101 NATURAL WAYS TO LOSE WEIGHT

Natural weight Loss: A Lifestyle, Not a Fad

LAUREN M. GREEN

DESCRIPTION

Losing weight is probably the most difficult problem that many of us face daily. Natural weight loss is preferable to fad or crash dieting programs. Fads and crash diets cause you to lose fluid and muscle tone first, which is why losing weight is so difficult. Weight loss can be achieved by altering your eating habits and increasing your physical activity. You don't have to do everything all at once. First, limit your chocolate bars to one or two per week rather than one or two every day. Smaller goals are easier to achieve than a large goal of twenty or thirty kilograms. Instead of keeping tempting ice cream in the freezer, be nice to yourself and go out for a treat.

Table of Contents

Introduction

Chapter One

Chapter Two

Chapter Three

Conclusion

Introduction

Losing weight is probably the most difficult problem that many of us face daily. Along with quitting smoking. It is one of the most difficult things to accomplish while remaining positive. Natural weight loss is preferable to fad or crash dieting programs. Fads and crash diets cause you to lose fluid and muscle tone first, which is why losing weight is so difficult. Weight loss can be achieved by altering your eating habits and increasing your physical activity. You don't have to accomplish everything all at once. First, restrict your chocolate bars to one or two per week rather than one or two per day. Smaller objectives are simpler to achieve than a large goal of twenty or thirty kg. Instead of keeping appealing ice cream in the freezer, be kind to yourself and go out for a treat.

Chapter One

Maintain a food journal.

Keeping a food diary is one of the simplest ways to monitor when and where you eat while trying to lose weight. When you reach a plateau and can't seem to lose any more weight or inches, write down everything you eat and drink every day to determine whether you're overeating at certain times of the day or if there's a way to adjust your eating habits. Some individuals like to have their major meal at midday and a smaller meal at night. The afternoon provides you with more time to put the energy from your meal to use.

Increase your physical activity.

Apart from eating less, exercise is the most effective approach to losing weight healthily.

There are several simple and fast methods to include extra exercise into your day.

- If feasible, walk to work, go to the next bus stop or get off one stop earlier.
- Use the stairs—even if you work on the tenth story, you can walk up a few floors every day.
- When you park your vehicle, make sure it is a considerable distance away from a shopping area which may also help you lose weight and become healthier.
- Join a walking club—many towns offer walking groups that stroll about town or travel to a central location and walk from there.
- Join a gym—some individuals like going to the gym, while others do not. If it fits your lifestyle, this might be a fantastic place to start with additional exercise.

- Obtaining a workout partner—it is usually simpler to exercise with someone else. On days when you don't feel like exercising, you can keep each other motivated.
- Play with the kids-kick a ball around in the park with the kids, shoot some hoops-it all adds up and you'll be shocked how much exercise you can get in half an hour of kicking a soccer ball.
- Walking the dog is usually a delight for them. Make a regular stroll or ball game in the park a habit.

Better shopping

Instead of packaged foods, go for fresh fruits and vegetables and unprocessed meals. Put it back on the shelf if it contains more than 5 ingredients or an ingredient you can't pronounce.

- Remove any packaged bakery items (cakes, biscuits, and cookies).
- Instead of cakes and pastries, choose fresh fruits and vegetables to nibble on.
- Shop on an empty stomach
- Make and stick to a shopping list.
- Be wary of low-fat substitutes; many low-fat foods have greater levels of sugar and salt. Many low-fat dairy products are loaded with sugar to mimic the flavour of full-fat items. It is generally preferable to consume less of the full-fat product and avoid the low-fat option.

Chapter Two

Change your eating habits

The underlisted tips are habits you need to incorporate into your eating.

- **Slow down while eating.**

Eating slowly allows your brain to recognize when you are full. You will discover that you can eat less while still feeling satisfied.

- **Consume breakfast**

Starting to eat breakfast every day is one of the most significant techniques to lose weight. Meal skipping is not a good method to reduce weight. Eat less, but eat more often.

- **Consume more fresh fruits and vegetables.**

The more colourful your fruits and veggies, the more vitamins and minerals you will acquire. Fruit includes antioxidants that are beneficial to human health, and it is present in colourful fruits such as blueberries.

- **Get rid of processed meals.**

Our processed meals are high in quick-acting carbs that are high in sugar, salt, and occasionally fat. Many baked items include trans fat, which is unhealthy. Olive oil and the natural fats found in lean meat are both beneficial to our health. They keep our joints healthy, and we require a certain amount each day.

- **Consume more fish.**

Oily fish is high in omega-3 fatty acids, which are beneficial to our health and assist to decrease cholesterol.

- **Consume more fibre.**

Fibre is the substance that keeps you fuller for longer periods and promotes bowel health. It aids in the removal of excess fat from the body and is an essential component of a healthy diet. If you don't think you're getting enough fibre, try adding oats to cereal, bran to your cereal, and dried peas and lentils to soups and vegetable dishes.

- **Include vegetarian dishes.**

Every week, eat a couple of vegetarian dishes. You'll be shocked at the range of meals you may prepare for the whole family.

Avoid meat alternatives in favour of eggs, and for protein, incorporate dry pulses or almonds. Replace a meat supper with a fresh salad of greens, fresh herbs, tomatoes, cucumber, celery, and olives.

- **Use probiotics.**

Probiotics are living microorganisms that provide health advantages when consumed. They may benefit digestive and cardiovascular health, and may even aid in weight reduction.

According to research, persons who are overweight or obese have different gut flora than normal-weight people, which may impact their weight.

Probiotics may aid in the regulation of healthy gut microorganisms. They may also inhibit dietary fat absorption while decreasing appetite and inflammation.

Lactobacillus gasseri is the probiotic bacterium with the most potential benefits for weight reduction.

- **Consume less meat.**

Reduce the amount of lean meat you consume. 2/3 to 34% of your plate should be veggies, with the remainder being lean protein. Meat is still vital for iron and other nutrients, but eating less red meat will make you feel less bloated. Red meat that is medium to rare is simpler to digest.

Consume less saturated fats.

Saturated fats may be present in processed and packaged meals and accumulate in our bodies as fat. These are the fats that contribute to heart disease by producing harmful cholesterol.

- **Avoid consuming liquid calories.**

Sugary soft drinks, fruit juices, chocolate milk, and energy drinks all include liquid calories.

These beverages are harmful to one's health in a variety of ways, including an increased risk of obesity. One research found that each daily consumption of a sugar-sweetened beverage increased the risk of childhood obesity by 60%.

It's also worth noting that your brain does not recognize liquid calories in the same way that it does solid calories, so you wind up piling these calories on top of everything else you consume.

- **Limit your intake of refined carbohydrates.**

Refined carbohydrates have had the majority of their essential elements and fibre removed.

The refining procedure produces only readily digestible carbohydrates, which might raise the risk of overeating and illness.

White flour, white bread, white rice, sodas, pastries, snacks, sweets, pasta, morning cereals, and added sugar are the most common dietary sources of refined carbohydrates.

- **Intermittent Fasting**

Intermittent fasting is an eating habit that alternates between fasting and eating intervals.

Intermittent fasting may be done in a variety of ways, including the 5:2 diet, the 16:8 approach, and the eat-stop-eat strategy.

In general, these approaches cause you to consume fewer calories overall, without having to intentionally limit calories during meal times. This should result in weight reduction as well as a slew of other health advantages.

- **Consume low-GI foods.**

Food with a lower GI keeps you fuller for longer since it takes your body longer to break it down. Most calorie counters contain a GI list, and many grocery goods, such as yoghurt, have a GI mentioned on the label.

- **Reduce the salt and increase the herbs and spices.**

Using less salt lowers blood pressure and prevents you from seeking unhealthy fizzy beverages, sodas, and cordials. To make your taste buds zing, add flavour to your cuisine using herbs and spices. When you add chili to your meals, it may boost your metabolism and help you lose weight.

- **Cut down on quick-acting carbs.**

By eliminating them from your diet, you will feel fuller for longer and have a decreased risk of developing diabetes. These carbs produce an increase in insulin levels, which raises blood sugar.

In soups, substitute barley and dry pulses such as lentils, split peas, kidney beans, borlotti beans, haricot beans, lima beans, or cannellini beans for rice and pasta.

- **Select grain bread with greater fibre content.**

Make a barley risotto with your favourite vegetables like mushrooms and asparagus, as well as some lean-cooked chicken or prawns.

- **Healthy beverages**

Include nutritious beverages in your diet. Water is wonderful, and sometimes when you are hungry, you are thirsty. So drink a glass of water and check whether you're still hungry. If you can't drink 2 litres of water every day, you can drink anything else.

- Iced tea-for a delightful drink, brew a litre of black tea, add lemon juice or mint leaves, and ice cubes.
- Green tea is an excellent beverage since it is high in antioxidants.
- Clear broth created from meat and vegetables—similar to preparing stock—can be flavoured with your favourite herbs and spices.

- **Choose from fat-releasing foods.**

Consume fat-releasing meals to avoid feeling starved and bingeing on higher-calorie items. Some foods aid in the removal of fat from our diets more than others, and they are healthy options. Protein, fibre, and vitamin C-rich foods are a wonderful place to start.

- Drizzle honey over natural yoghurt and fresh fruit for just 64 fat-releasing calories per tablespoon.

- Eggs are low in calories and high in fat-releasing protein. To make it even more attractive, sprinkle it with chives.
- Ricotta is cheese-free, the low-fat only 39 calories in one ounce of this food, packed with fat-releasing calcium For dessert, spoon over a dish of fresh fruit.
- A one-ounce square of dark chocolate has around 168 calories, but it contains high levels of fat-releasing fibre.
- 12 big shrimp-good omega oils and just 60 calories

- **Get Enough Rest**

Getting adequate sleep is critical for weight reduction and preventing future weight gain.

Sleep-deprived persons are up to 55% more likely to acquire obese than those who receive adequate sleep, according to studies.

This figure is significantly greater among children.

This is due, in part, to the fact that sleep deprivation affects the daily oscillations in hunger hormones, resulting in poor appetite control.

- **Eat more at home.**

When you dine at home, you have more control over who is on your plate and are less likely to be enticed by rich creamy sauces and calorie-laden sweets. You may always go out to eat as a treat, but you may discover that the food is too heavy and fatty for you, making you feel bloated and nauseated. If you want takeout on occasion, pick intelligently and make smarter choices.

- Salads with oil-free dressings are available.

- Say goodbye to creamy dressings and mayonnaise.
- Choose a pizza without cheese or one with low-fat cheese.

Eat less often.

- **Make use of a smaller plate.**

Instead of a dinner plate, serve your meal on a bread and butter plate. As your plate fills up, it seems that you are eating more. It defeats the point if you pile your old-size food on the platter. It does not seem like you are limiting yourself by eating less and using a smaller dish.

- **5 Simple meals every day.**

Use a smaller plate and eat five little meals every day.

- You will never feel hungry and will never overeat.
- Divide your calories across the five meals.
- Start your day with a larger breakfast.

- **Eat Healthy snacks.**

To stay at home, only purchase healthy foods.

- Frozen yoghurt may be used instead of ice cream.
- Raw nuts may be used instead of crisps.
- Make your butter-free popcorn.
- Make a salad with fresh veggies and a delightful no-oil dressing. Lettuces, red, green, and yellow peppers, spring onions or shallots, carrot and celery sticks, and sliced mushrooms are also available.

Chapter Three

Set Goals

Set goals for yourself that you can attain. Don't make losing weight your only objective. Divide it into manageable chunks. Try to drop 10 kg at a time, starting with minor targets to gradually improve your eating habits. If you establish objectives for yourself that you believe you can attain with a little additional work, you will find yourself exceeding them and creating new ones. Don't be too ambitious and set impossible objectives for yourself; you'll wind up feeling disheartened and unhappy, giving up, and reverting to your previous eating habits. It all comes down to eating the appropriate meals and neither starving yourself nor exercising like a madman and being ill to achieve that objective.

Food

- With coffee, one fewer biscuit
- A slice of fruit per day
- Dinner should include a colourful vegetable.
- fewer cups of coffee
- Remove one item at a time.

Exercise

- Every day, take a walk around the block.
- Every week, do some gardening.
- On weekends, take the dog for a walk.
- Every day, add 10 minutes of exercise.
- Purchase a pedometer and walk 1000 steps every day.

Eating

- Every day, eat breakfast.

- Every day, eat three meals and two snacks.
- At night, use a smaller dish for supper.
- Slow down and enjoy the flavour of your food.
- Don't eat in front of the TV.

The Influence of Positive Thinking.

Never undervalue the power of optimistic thinking. It might improve your mood and help you lose weight faster. Begin with loving yourself, regardless of size. Find anything you appreciate about yourself, whether it's your long hair, your eyes, your ankles, or your legs. Whatever it is, make your bad obesity a good aspect of yourself. There are methods to be optimistic.

- Find a mantra that you like and repeat it numerous times every day. "I will lose weight," "I am becoming healthier," and "I am feeling better."
- Make time each day to meditate or sit quietly by yourself. Concentrate on yourself rather than your spouse or children. This will also help you sleep better.

Conclusion

Losing weight naturally will never be simple or quick, but you will gradually reduce weight, feel better, and see the story in a new light. You won't feel like you're on a diet if you change a few parts of your lifestyle at a time. You are beginning to eat healthier and exercise more, and as a result, you are losing weight.

It will be easier to exercise with a partner to provide motivation and encouragement. A person who exercises with a companion will push themselves even harder. So instead of going on a diet, choose a healthy eating plan to become fitter and stronger.